George H. Constantine, PhD

Tyler's Tips
The Shopper's Guide for Herbal Remedies

Pre-publication REVIEWS, COMMENTARIES, EVALUATIONS . . .

"**B**otanical dietary supplements or phytomedicines have become very popular in the United States over the past ten years. Some estimates state that over seventy million Americans use herbal products on a regular basis. Since there is very little FDA control of the botanical dietary supplement industry, a plethora of products from innumerable manufacturers has flooded the market as public interest and demand have increased. At the moment, the general public is bewildered by the vast array of products to choose from. *Tyler's Tips* offers a wonderful guide for those shoppers who desire some degree of knowledge before purchasing an herbal product. The commonly used herbs are arranged in this convenient pocket book according to the particular health condition to be addressed. Each herb is approached in the same fashion, which facilitates consumer understanding. Very practical information on herbal product use is presented in an easy to understand, condensed format. This book is a must for those herbal consumers who desire a knowledge base before making a purchase. An excellent household reference for the commonly used phytomedicines written by a highly qualified pharmacognosist."

William L. Keller, PhD
*Professor and Chair,
Department of Pharmaceutical
Sciences, Samford University,
Birmingham, AL*

Tyler's Tips
The Shopper's Guide for Herbal Remedies

Tyler's Tips
The Shopper's Guide for Herbal Remedies

George H. Constantine, PhD

The Haworth Herbal Press
An Imprint of The Haworth Press, Inc.
New York • London • Oxford

Published by

The Haworth Herbal Press, an imprint of the The Haworth Press, Inc., 10 Alice Street, Binghamton, NY 13904-1580

Medicine is an ever-changing science. As new research and clinical experience broaden our knowledge, changes in treatment and drug therapy are required. While many suggestions for drug usages are made herein, the book is intended for educational purposes only, and the author, editor, and publisher do not accept liability in the event of negative consequences incurred as a result of information presented in this book. We do not claim that this information is necessarily accurate by the rigid, scientific standard applied for medical proof, and therefore make no warranty, expressed or implied, with respect to the material herein contained. Therefore the patient is urged to check the product information sheet included in the package of each drug he or she plans to administer to be certain the protocol followed is not in conflict with the manufacturer's inserts. When a discrepancy arises between these inserts and information in this book, the physician is encouraged to use his or her best professional judgement.

Cover design by Jennifer M. Gaska.

Library of Congress Cataloging-in-Publication Data

Constantine, George H.
 Tyler's tips : the shopper's guide for herbal remedies / George H. Constantine.
  p. cm.
 "A guide to the most effective and safe herbal products and their proper use as identified by Varro E. Tyler, Ph.D., Dean and Distinguished Professor Emeritus, Purdue University."
 Includes bibliographical references and index.
 ISBN 0-7890-0948-X (hardcover : alk. paper) — ISBN 0-7890-0949-8 (soft : alk. paper)
 1. Herbs—Therapeutic use. I. Tyler, Varro E. II. Title.

RM666.H33 .C68 2000
615'.321—dc21

00-039706

To Mom and Dad, who taught me to enjoy
science, philosophy, and life,

To Nancy, who made all these enjoyments
possible and much more, and

To my friends and colleagues in the
American Society of Pharmacognosy.

ABOUT THE AUTHOR

George H. Constantine, PhD, is Professor Emeritus of Pharmacognosy and Drug Information at the College of Pharmacy, Oregon State University at Corvallis, where his responsibilities include student recruitment, retention, advising, public relations, fund raising, curriculum development, alumni/university relations, and long-range planning. He has taught courses in natural products chemistry, alternative medicine, antimicrobial chemotherapy, endocrinology, drug abuse, medical ethics, gerontology, and drug information.

Dr. Constantine has served as a consultant on herbal remedies to the Oregon State Board of Pharmacy and Board of Medical Examiners and is the co-founder of Benton Hospice in Corvallis, Oregon.

CONTENTS

SECTION V: HERBAL REMEDIES TO AID PROSTATE HEALTH

SECTION VI: HERBAL REMEDIES TO AID WEIGHT LOSS

SECTION VII: HERBAL REMEDIES TO ALLEVIATE HEADACHE/PAIN

SECTION VIII: HERBAL REMEDIES TO ALLEVIATE CONSTIPATION

SECTION IX: HERBAL REMEDIES TO ALLEVIATE LIVER DYSFUNCTION

SECTION X: HERBAL REMEDIES TO ALLEVIATE BLADDER PROBLEMS

SECTION XI: HERBAL REMEDIES TO ALLEVIATE ULCERS AND INTESTINAL PROBLEMS

SECTION XII: HERBAL REMEDIES TO ALLEVIATE SKIN PROBLEMS AND EXTERNAL SORES

Preface

Shopper's Guide to Herbal Products

INTRODUCTION

This guide is intended to be used by those who wish to use herbal products for a variety of different conditions and may not be aware of all the products that are available for use. In this volume, the products are found in different therapeutic categories.

The coverage of the conditions is extensive, but consideration will be limited to those popular plants that have a lengthy history of use and/or documented scientific evidence for their safety and effectiveness.

The primary sources of information are the following:

Herbal Drugs and Phytopharmaceuticals, edited by M. Wichtl (German) N. Bassett (English), 1994, CRC Press, Boca Raton, Florida.

Rational Phytotherapy: A Physician's Guide to Herbal Medicine, V. Schultz, R. Hänsel, and V.E. Tyler, 1998, Springer-Verlag, New York.

The Review of Natural Products, B. Olin, ed., Facts and Comparisons, St. Louis, Missouri (a subscription monograph series).

Tyler's Herbs of Choice, Second Edition, by James E. Robbers and Varro E. Tyler, 1999, The Haworth Herbal Press, Binghamton, New York.

Tyler's Honest Herbal, Fourth Edition, Steven Foster and Varro E. Tyler, 1998, The Haworth Herbal Press, Binghamton, New York.

The secondary sources are the following:

The Complete Guide to Herbs, S. Bratman, 1999, Prima Publishing, Rocklin, California.

The Green Pharmacy, J.A. Duke, 1998, St. Martin's paperbacks, New York.

A Manual of Materia Medica and Pharmacology, D.M.R. Culbreth, 1917, Lea and Febiger, New York.

Physicians' Desk Reference, 1999, Medical Economics, Montvale, New Jersey.

The United States Dispensatory, G.B. Wood and F. Bache, 1845, Grigg and Elliot, Philadelphia.

Plants As Medicines and Now Dietary Supplements

Since ancient times, the plant kingdom has been used as a source of food, shelter, and for medical and religious purposes. The ancient Egyptians, Greeks, Romans, and Chinese all have a long history of using plants. Unfortunately, many of the original sources of this information are no longer available. What is available has furnished modern medicine with clues to the uses of plants in the past and how their constituents could be developed as medicines.

In the United States, the use of plants as medicines is verified by a review of the first *United States Pharmacopoeia* (USP) published in 1820. Over 80 percent of the medicines described therein were of plant origin, although most were dropped by the mid-twentieth century. Ironically, in 1998, the USP again began publishing plant monographs.

The surge of interest during the past decade increased enormously when the U.S. Congress passed the Dietary Supplement and Health Education Act (DSHEA) in 1994. This Act allows herbal preparations to be defined as dietary supplements and not medicines or drugs. They are not required to meet any safety or efficacy standards as are all over-the-counter medicines.

Sales of herbal preparations have grown astronomically in the past five years, both in the United States and Europe, where herbal products have long been traditional. European manufacturers in Germany must meet standards for products to be sold as drugs. To date, that same practice has not occurred in this country, however, it is slowly evolving.

In the meantime, purchasers of herbal products in the United States need to know that these products may or may not contain ingredients that are stated on the labels. Until such a time when there are mandatory standards of quality, all a purchaser can do is to continue buying from a manufacturer whose product has been proven to be useful. In contrast, if one product from one manufacturer is ineffective, this does not mean that a similar product from another manufacturer will also be ineffective.

PRECAUTIONS AND DISCLAIMERS

Most people consider an herb to be safe and effective just because it is classified as a natural dietary supplement. One has only to briefly review the literature available in any library or Internet site to locate huge volumes of information on poisonous plants and mushrooms. None of the plants covered in this guide have ever been reported to produce any severe toxic effects in normal usage. The reader must always be aware that contamination by herbicides, pesticides, and other substances can occur. Unfortunately, some herbal producers, especially in Asia, have purposely added prescription drugs to their products to increase their biological activity. A prime example is the addition of the potent anti-inflammatory Butazolidin to several Chinese herbal products. Only when reports of gastrointestinal upsets appeared did this come to the attention of the public.

Proper Identification

Most processors and vendors of herbal products have some type of quality control system whereby they can accurately identify an herb by either botanical identification or the contents of one or more active or marker compounds in the plant. Once again, there have been several instances of some irresponsible companies not doing so and then including a poisonous plant in a product (e.g., plantain leaves contaminated with similar appearing Grecian foxglove leaves), or of people collecting their own plants in the wild.

Proper Plant Part

Recent trends indicate that some producers of herbal products are using a part of the plant that has very little, if any, history of use. A case in point is the purple coneflower (*Echinacea* spp.). The German Commission E approved the roots of *E. pallida* (Nutt.) Nutt. and the tops of *E. purpurea* (L.) Moench. Some producers are now using both the roots and tops of these two plants plus *E. angustifolia* DC. in all sorts of combinations. Many of these combinations have never been tested clinically and vendors are now selling all parts of these three species with very little documentation that they contain the same biological activity as the approved products. Many medicinal plants are well-known for having a wide variation in concentrations of biologically active substances depending on their location in the plant.

Proper Preparation and Subsequent Storage

Not only should the herbal processor take proper precautions in assuring quality during preparation of dosage forms, but the ultimate user should also assume some responsibility for storage when the product is taken home. Most powdered plant materials should be stored in a dry, cool location away from direct light, preferably in airtight containers. For example, the reputed active compound in feverfew, parthenolide, is very unstable. Some manufacturers are now placing expiration dates on the labels, but until the active ingredients are known and their stability determined, this may be totally useless information.

Untoward or Adverse Reactions

Almost any foreign object, whether it be a chemical, an insect, a pollen, etc., can produce an allergic response. Depending on the location in the body, the intensity of the reaction caused, and the length of exposure, the body may respond in a variety of unpleasant ways, ranging from minor sniffles to severe heart malfunction. If these reactions are minor and can be relieved by withdrawal of the offending material, they are usually referred to as untoward reactions. However, serious adverse reactions may require invasive medical attention in lifesaving situations. Fortunately, to date, there have been limited reports of toxicity when herbs are used properly. Fatalities or the need for organ transplants due to liver toxicity have usually been associated with persons who, for purposes of weight loss, consumed excessive quantities of teas containing known toxic plants such as germander or comfrey. Stephania and magnolia teas have caused kidney failure, and comfrey root in capsules has produced liver toxicity. Once again, it is essential that proper dosing be followed with all herbal products. Although herbs are legally classified as dietary supplements (foods), technically they are drugs and must be treated with respect.

Interactions with Other Foods or Other Medicines

A major cause for concern among health professionals is the question of drug-drug, drug-food, or herb-drug interactions. The amount of information published in the medical literature documenting serious interactions is very limited. Some of this lack may be due to nonreporting since persons admitted to an emergency room may not disclose to the medical staff their use of an herbal remedy. Another reason might be that even if the staff is notified, they may be unaware that this should be reported in the same fashion as any other adverse effect, i.e., report to the manufacturer as well as the FDA (see herb-drug interactions). As with anything that we place in the body, the potential exists for herbs to react with other substances, particularly any medications that are being taken for possible life-threatening conditions, e.g., high blood pressure, diabetes, and even some cancers.

Most herb-drug interactions can be avoided by using common sense. Do not take St. John's wort at the same time as a prescription antidepressant unless the combination is advised by a qualified physician. Do not use kava and Valium or similar medicines at the same time. Do not use herbs that prolong blood clotting time, such as ginkgo, with medicines that have the same effects, e.g., Coumadin. Do not take phytoestrogens if you have a family history of breast or cervical cancer.

Self-Diagnosis

Before using an herbal preparation of any kind, individuals should ascertain that the signs and symptoms of the condition do not represent a major disease. The potential consumer should have an accurate diagnosis from a competent medical practitioner before embarking on self-treatment.

The potential for misuse arises in the following situations:

1. Treatment of an assumed prostate problem when a cancerous condition may be present.
2. Treating a menopausal symptom with herbs containing "phytoestrogens," which may cause the same adverse effects as synthetic estrogens, e.g., excess estrogen-dependent

cell growth in the breast or uterus, interactions with anti-cancer agents that are antiestrogens, etc.

3. Treating a urinary tract infection that could be a more serious kidney infection.

4. Treating a heart condition that could be a sign or symptom of a truly serious problem.

5. Treatment of tiredness or fatigue that could be caused by a variety of factors, ranging from a poor diet to severe depression.

6. Treating a local skin infection with a topical remedy when a systemic agent may perform more effectively.

7. Treating the potentially debilitating effects of osteoporosis by means other than diet, exercise, calcium supplementation, or proven prescription medicines.

8. Treating a constant sore throat with gargles or washes when a viral or bacterial infection, such as *Strep*, could be the culprit; or treating local fungal infections with an ineffective product, one to which the causative organism is not susceptible. (More than eight species of fungi can cause fungal infections and twelve or more can cause systemic infections.)

9. Treating diabetes, particularly the adult-obese type, which can often be controlled with diet and exercise, or oral medications if warranted. Remember, many herbs may lower blood sugar, but none are standardized to produce a uniform effect.

Although the above list is incomplete, consumers should make certain that the condition being treated is not suggestive of a more serious condition. Once an appropriate diagnosis is made and herbal use has begun, use the herb only until the condition is relieved. If the condition is long lasting, one may ordinarily continue if no adverse effects are encountered. However, in some cases, specific limitations have been established by authorities. These can be found in the pages that follow.

PURPOSE OF THIS BOOK

In this book, readers will be able to locate accurate and precise summaries of information on a wide variety of herbs that have been evaluated (tested) and shown to have positive results by appropriate scientific and clinical studies. The details presented are *not* based mainly on folklore, gossip, or testimonials by over-ambitious salespersons.

Each herb description contains information on the constituents in the plants that are usually measured to ensure a uniformly effective dose. All herbs contain one or more compounds that are responsible for their effects on the body. If the compound is known to be effective, it is an "active" ingredient, if not, some other compound can be measured and is used as a "marker." This "marker" then can be measured to ensure that the plant being used is the proper one as specified on the label.

Acknowledgments

Grateful thanks are extended to Dr. Varro E. Tyler for offering the opportunity to compile this shopping guide. His trust, mentoring, and comments have been invaluable.

Denise Hoffmann performed minor miracles by constantly accepting modifications of many drafts of the manuscript. Her competence and devotion to this work deserves the highest praise.

PhD candidate Ken Milligan (Oregon State University), a friend and a very thorough and meticulous reviewer of this manuscript, spent hours ensuring that the final draft was without significant flaws.

Ruben Gonzales-Loredo, PhD (University of Durango-Mexico), friend and astute "typo-expert" helped to ensure quality control.

Chris Meletis, ND (National College of Naturopathic Medicine, Portland), graciously supplied the majority of the price information on quality herbal products that are used in his practice as chief of clinics. I am sincerely grateful for his efforts.

SECTION I:
HERBAL REMEDIES
TO AID MENTAL HEALTH

St. John's Wort
Hypericum perforatum L.

Condensed Facts:

One of the best-researched herbal products with over 3,000 people having achieved positive results in well-conducted clinical trials.

Conditions:

Used for mild to moderate, *not* severe, depression. May be useful for anxiety and seasonal affective disorder.

Plants/Standard:

Hypericum perforatum is found in the wild in Europe, Asia, and North and South America. This herb, in most products that contain it, is cultivated in order to ensure a standard product.

What to Look For:

Hypericin is used as a "marker" compound, although it is not the only active ingredient. Most products are standardized to 0.3 percent hypericin, but even this quantity is not assured (one study confirmed that only two of eight products approach this concentration*). Some more recent products are now being standardized to 3 to 5 percent hyperforin.

Traditional Dosing/ Dosage Forms:

Most European clinical studies used 900 mg/day, the usual recommended dosage of products found in the United States. The active chemicals will degrade on exposure to light, so store them properly.

Actions/Uses:

This herb is effective in treating mild to moderate depression, anxiety, and perhaps seasonal affective disorder.

Precautions:

Fewer than 3 percent of over 3,000 treatment cases showed any side effects. Excessive sunburn reactions may occur in fair-skinned people, but this is rare with normal doses. Combining *Hypericum perforatum* with other antidepressant medication is not recommended unless done so under the direction of a qualified physician.

Typical Price:

Tincture, 1 oz = $9.00
Capsules = $9.50/45 - $13.50/60
Powder, 1 oz = $3.00

---

*G. H. Constantine and J. Karchesy, "Variations in hypericin concentrations in *Hypericum perforatum* L. and commercial preparations," *Journal of Pharmaceutical Biology 36*(5) 365-367 (1998).

Kava
Piper methysticum Forest. f.

Condensed Facts: The use of kava as a ceremonial beverage was observed by Captain Cook in his voyages to the South Seas. By 1966, most of the active compounds (kavapyrones or kavalactones) had been identified and some are now made synthetically.

Conditions: Kava can be used for anxiety and insomnia. The action on the body is similar to the benzodiazepine drugs (Librium, Valium, etc.) but without causing dependency or mental cloudiness. It may be useful in higher doses as a muscle relaxant.

Plants/Standard: The active chemicals are not water soluble. The ground rhizomes are used and extracted with either water/alcohol or acetone/water.

What to Look For: The dried herb should contain 3.5 percent kavapyrones (kawain).

Traditional Dosing/ Dosage Forms: Most clinical studies used extracts containing 70 percent kavapyrones in doses equivalent to 60 to 210 mg of these active principles.

5

Actions/Uses: Kava produces antianxiety effects
                           similar to that of some prescription
                           drugs.

Precautions: Should not be combined with alco-
                           hol, other tranquilizers, or sedatives.
                           Very few side effects at usual doses,
                           mainly stomach or allergic reactions
                           (1 to 2.3 percent). Long-term use
                           may produce a dry, scaly skin and/or
                           a yellowish discoloration of the skin.

Typical Price: Tincture, 1 oz = $9.00
                           Capsules = $9.50/45 - $14.90/60
                           Powder, 1 oz = $2.50

Ginkgo
Ginkgo biloba L.

Condensed Facts: The ginkgo tree has existed on earth for 300 million years. Its seeds, not the leaves, were used in traditional Chinese medicine.

Conditions: Ginkgo is primarily used for various cognitive deficiencies, such as early-stage Alzheimer's disease and other declines in memory or mental function. In Europe, it is also used for people who have poor leg circulation, dizziness, or ringing in the ears. One small study has shown benefits in relieving impotence caused by antidepressant drugs.

Plants/Standard: Ginkgo leaf extracts are available as tinctures and in capsules, tablets, and now even soft drinks and teas.

What to Look For: Quality products consist of an extract standardized to contain 24 percent ginkgo-flavone glycosides and 6 percent terpene lactones. This represents a fifty-fold concentration of the leaf.

Traditional Dosing/ Dosage Forms: More than forty clinical studies of over 2,000 patients evaluating the uses of ginkgo for dementia patients used 120 to 240 mg/day. This is the usual dosage range.

Actions/Uses: Ginkgo is documented to benefit patients with age-related mental deterioration. Increased walking distances have been documented when ginkgo was given to patients with inadequate circulation in the legs (intermittent claudication).

Precautions: About 1.7 percent of the thousands of patients taking ginkgo suffered side effects; nausea and headaches were the most common. (Compare this to 5.4 percent reported with prescription medicines used for the same purpose.) A few cases of bleeding disorders have been reported recently. Consequently, care should be taken if other blood-thinning herbs, vitamins (vitamin E), or medicines (warfarin, aspirin, etc.) are taken at the same time.

Typical Price: Tincture, 1 oz = $9.00
Capsules = $9.50/45 - $14.30/60
Powder, 1 oz = $2.00

Other Herbals for Potential Use to Aid Mental Health

VALERIAN (*Valeriana officinalis* L.)

Over 250 species exist but only the root of *V. officinalis* has been clinically evaluated; others may be less potent and/or more toxic. Used primarily as a treatment for insomnia and as a mild tranquilizer. Tablets (coated) are now available because the dried herb or liquid extract has an unpleasant odor. Capsules are also available. Products usually contain 2 to 3 grams of dried root per dose or extracts with equivalent amounts.

LEMON BALM (*Melissa officinalis*)

A fragrant lemon-like tea has a mild relaxing effect and is used to induce sleep. It also alleviates gastrointestinal disorders. Recently, studies in Europe have shown that ointments containing *Melissa* are effective in treating oral and genital herpes.

PASSION FLOWER (*Passiflora incarnata*)

No definitive studies, but traditional use holds that some preparations may be effective in alleviating restlessness, mild sleeping difficulties, and gastrointestinal disorders.

Herbal Benefits of Remedies
to Aid Mental Health

The roots of *Rauvolfia serpentina* were used in India for years prior to the discovery that its active principle, reserpine, could be used to treat anxiety and high blood pressure. It was the first significant antipsychotic agent. Unfortunately, it produced undesirable side effects, including: gastritis, leading to ulcers; dizziness; respiratory difficulty; skin irritation; joint and muscular pain; frequent bowel movements; increased weight. In higher doses it caused cardiac depression, insomnia, despondency, and suicidal tendencies.

From that beginning, a wide range of agents became available to treat anxiety (Librium, Serax, Xanax), to use as anti-depressants (Desyrel, Serzone, Wellbutrin), to treat mood disorders (Elavil, Sinequan, Etrafon) and to treat mixed disorders (Paxil, Prozac, Zoloft). All of these agents have greatly assisted many people and made the public aware that many mental conditions are treatable.

The addition of the readily available *Hypericum* for mild to moderate depression adds a useful herb to the above menu. None of the prescription products can report such a low incidence of side effects or a lack of reported drug interactions. Kava also offers another effective natural product for the treatment of anxiety.

SECTION II:
HERBAL REMEDIES
TO AID THE IMMUNE SYSTEM

Echinacea
Echinaceae pallida (Nutt.) Nutt.,
E. purpurea (L.) Moench,
or *E. angustifolia* DC.

Condensed Facts:

The purple coneflower was used by many Midwestern Native American tribes for a wide range of conditions, ranging from sore eyes to snake bites.

Conditions:

Marketed in Europe for the treatment of colds and flu (root extracts of *E. angustifolia* and *E. pallida,* or the pressed juice for the above-ground parts of *E. purpurea*) and to support and promote natural resistance due to infections.

Plants/Standard:

All three plants and their extracts are assumed to be similar, but few studies have documented this fact. The active compounds include complex polysaccharides, alkamides, and cichoric acid and its derivatives. Although many products are standardized on the basis of phenolic constituents, no truly useful standards on the basis of active constituents have been established.

What to Look For:	Teas, tablets, capsules, expressed juice, and tinctures. At least forty different branded products are available. Dosages vary greatly depending on the method of preparation, plant and plant part used, etc. Follow the instructions on the label.
Traditional Dosing/ Dosage Forms:	A quality product should contain the equivalent of 900 mg of the crude drug per daily dose. European experts state that echinacea should not be taken continuously for more than eight weeks.
Actions/Uses:	Reducing duration and severity of symptoms of colds and flu, and helping the body fight infections. Can also be used topically.
Precautions:	Some people may be sensitive to daisy plants, but no other significant adverse effects have been reported.
Typical Price:	Varies greatly depending on source, type of product, and product strength. Capsules = $9.50/45 - $14.00/50 Powder, 1 oz = $2.50

Astragalus Root
Astragalus membranaceous

Condensed Facts:

A root herb used in traditional Chinese medicine (TCM) to strengthen immunity.

Conditions:

In contrast to echinacea, astragalus is assumed to strengthen the immune system prior to, not during, an infection. Astragalus has reportedly benefited a wide spectrum of conditions, from high blood pressure to AIDS. These have not been verified by significant clinical studies.

Plants/Standard:

Astragalus root can be found in many Chinese formula products or as the dried herb.

What to Look For:

Depend on the label since there is no standard established for any of the compounds that may be responsible for the biological effects.

Traditional Dosing/ Dosage Forms:

From 9 to 30 grams of the dried root is used to make a tea. As with all TCM remedies, this may be combined with as many as twelve other herbs.

Actions/Uses: Said to stimulate the immune sys-
                                 tem, it may have other unproven
                                 medical benefits.

Precautions: None known.

Typical Price: Tincture, 1 oz = $9.00
                                 Capsules, 90 = $10.50
                                 Powder, 1 oz = $2.40

Herbal Benefits of Remedies to Aid the Immune System

Much research is being conducted worldwide on specific substances to stimulate the body's immune response, especially in the area of cancer therapy. While the herbals mentioned in this section have not been studied for this specific use, they are presently categorized as relatively mild, nonspecific immune stimulants.

Most data to date obtained from twenty-six reliable clinical studies on echinacea show positive effects, particularly for upper respiratory tract infections. Whether this herb has additional beneficial effects awaits additional research.

SECTION III:
TONICS (ADAPTOGENS)

Ginseng
Panax ginseng C. A. Meyer,
P. quinquefolius L.,
or *P. pseudo-ginseng* Wallich

Condensed Facts: Used in Asia for well over 2,000 years. Ginseng has been studied more extensively than any other medicinal plant.

Conditions: Mood improvement and mental and physical performance may be increased. It may positively effect fat and carbohydrate blood levels.

Plants/Standard: *P. ginseng* and *P. quinquefolius* are both cultivated in Asia and the United States. It takes six years or more to mature. There are many varieties; some people have a preference for white versus red. The color depends on the way the root is cured.

What to Look For: Ginseng roots contain 2 to 3 percent of active compounds known as ginsenosides. Commercial products vary considerably. Aside from dried roots, ginseng can now be found in tablets, capsules, teas, soft drinks, cosmetics, etc. Concentrations in cosmetics are almost never specified and may be insignificant.

**Traditional Dosing/
Dosage Forms:**

For preparing a tea, use 1 teaspoonful of chopped root (3 grams). Extracts containing 4 to 7 percent ginsenosides were used in studies at doses of 200 to 600 mg/day. It is generally suggested that it not be taken continually, but stop consumption for two to three weeks after use of up to three months.

Actions/Uses:

Many exaggerated claims have been made for ginseng, but the good studies that have been done indicate that it can improve mood, physical and intellectual performance, and may have positive effects on carbohydrate and fat metabolism.

Precautions:

No significant toxicity. Chinese herbalists do not advise use by pregnant women or nursing mothers.

Typical Price:

Considerable variation, but remember that ginseng is one of the most expensive herbs.

Eleuthero

Eleutherococcus senticosus
(Rupr. & Maxim.) Maxim.

Condensed Facts: Also known as Siberian ginseng. Promoted to be similar to true ginseng, eleuthero is much less expensive and does not contain active principles identical to those found in ginseng.

Conditions: Promoted as a ginseng product, but it is not. Studies performed in the 1960s in the former Soviet Union made claims that are questionable due to design weaknesses.

Plants/Standard: Eleuthero is a shrub of Siberia and Northern China. No standards available.

What to Look For: Inexpensive ginseng products should be suspected of containing Siberian ginseng. Look at the label to see if it says *Panax* or *Eleuthero*. Also, Chinese silk vine (*Periploca sepium* Bunge) is often substituted for eleuthero. Purchase only from a reliable source.

Traditional Dosing/ Dosage Forms: For a tea, 2 to 3 grams of chopped or 300 or 400 mg of extract/day.

Actions/Uses: Reportedly for same purposes as *Panax*.

Precautions: Not recommended in cases of high blood pressure.

Typical Price: Varies considerably.

Ashwagandha
Withania somnifera Dunal

Condensed Facts:	The root of this plant has been used in Indian traditional medicine (Ayurvedic) for years, primarily for uses similar to ginseng with more emphasis on its use for male fertility.
Conditions:	This herbal has had limited exposure in the United States, but recently it has received increased attention for use as a sexual stimulant and fertility remedy.
Plants/Standard:	Only the root product should be used. No standards on active compounds.
What to Look For:	Powdered root material is of limited availability, but it can be found in locations that sell Indian traditional medicines, often in combination with other herbs.
Traditional Dosing/ Dosage Forms:	One teaspoonful of powdered root as a tea. No standard established.
Actions/Uses:	General tonic (stimulant) qualities.
Precautions:	None known.
Typical Price:	Not usually available as a single herb (see above).

Other Herbals
for Potential Use As Tonics

MAITAKE (*Grifola frondosa*)

This mushroom has been used in Japan as a health promoter. Claims range from curing cancer and preventing heart disease, to treating AIDS, diabetes, and high cholesterol. No substantial studies done to date.

REISHI (*Ganoderma lucidum*)

This tree fungus is now being cultivated and consequently is available in food and health stores. As with maitake, it has many claims for medicinal use, but there is a significant lack of definitive human clinical trials to support the claims.

SUMA [*Pfaffia paniculata* (Mart.) Kuntze.]

This vine from South America has been referred to as "Brazilian ginseng." Once again, there are many anecdotal reports, especially about the aphrodisiac qualities, but human clinical trials to support these claims are lacking.

Herbal Benefits of Tonics

Aside from proper diet on one extreme to steroids on the other, no other products come close to the effects of the herbal tonics. Ginseng has many positive qualities documented by human clinical trials. Unfortunately, some people who sell these products have made exaggerated and undocumented claims for other uses, and product quality for this expensive herb is often questionable.

SECTION IV:
HERBAL REMEDIES
TO ALLEVIATE MENOPAUSE
AND MENSTRUAL PROBLEMS

Black Cohosh
Cimicifuga racemosa (L.) Nutt.

Condensed Facts: A native North American plant used by Native Americans for a variety of disorders. It was once commonly used in America as an ingredient in the famous proprietary medicine, Lydia E. Pinkham's "Vegetable Compound."

Conditions: Used for treating all menopausal conditions and symptoms.

Plants/Standard: Products should contain 40 mg/day of the dried roots and rhizomes.

What to Look For: Remifemin, a German trademark product, is available; it contains 1 mg of 27-deoxyactein. Tinctures and capsules are also available.

Traditional Dosing/ Dosage Forms: One or two Remifemin tablets/day. Capsules and tinctures should contain the equivalent of 40 mg of the dried plant.

Actions/Uses: Apparently functions by depressing the levels of a luteinizing hormone that rises during menopause. There are distinct improvements in the reduction of hot flashes, sweating, headache, dizziness, heart palpitations, ringing in the ears, nervousness, irritability, sleep disorders, anxiety, and depression. No evidence indicates that black cohosh can prevent osteoporosis or heart disease, conditions which estrogens can benefit.

Precautions:

Mild side effects such as stomach complaints, headache, and weight gain have been reported. Does not simulate breast cancer cells in a test tube but no large studies have been done to determine if this effect occurs in humans. Should not be used by adolescents and pregnant or nursing women.

Typical Price:

Tincture, 1 oz = $9.00
Capsules, 90 = $15.00 (Remifemin)

Chasteberry
Vitex angus-castus L.

Condensed Facts:	A Mediterranean shrub used as a medicinal plant for over 2,000 years. It was reportedly used by medieval monks to reduce sexual desire, therefore called monk's pepper.
Conditions:	Used primarily for PMS symptoms.
Plants/Standard:	Extracts of the berries have not been standardized but do demonstrate a decrease in the amount of prolactin, a pituitary hormone, in both rats and in human clinical trials.
What to Look For:	An extract or powdered, dried ripe fruits is used. No standard has been established.
Traditional Dosing/ Dosage Forms:	According to the German Commission E, 30 to 40 mg/day is required. Of the few clinical studies that have been done, some have used doses as high as 480 mg.
Actions/Uses:	May take at least eight to ten weeks to demonstrate effectiveness for treatment of PMS symptoms.
Precautions:	No significant side effects. Not to be used during pregnancy or while nursing.

Typical Price: Tincture, 1 oz = $9.00
                                       Capsules, 60 (225 mg each)
                                       = $9.50 - $16.95

Dong Quai
Angelica sinensis (Oliv.) Diels

Condensed Facts: Long used in Chinese medicine, this *Angelica* species is used primarily for menstrual disorders. The European plant, *A. archangelica* L., is used primarily to stimulate gastric and pancreatic secretions.

Conditions: Menstrual disorders and PMS symptoms.

Plants/Standard: Roots from plants at least three years old are used. No standard chemical or marker compounds have been identified.

What to Look For: Finely cut or powdered root material is used.

Traditional Dosing/Dosage Forms: Take one teaspoonful of tea (1.5 grams), tincture, or capsules. Often found in combination with other herbs with similar actions.

Actions/Uses: The only Western clinical trials failed to show any improvement in menopausal symptoms, but it has a long history of use in China.

Precautions: Some constituents may cause photosensitivity, so beware of excessive sun exposure.

Typical Price: Tincture, 1 oz = $9.00
                                      Capsules, 90 = $10.99
                                      Herbal teas prepared by a qualified
                                      Chinese herbalist. Price varies.

Red Clover
Trifolium pratense L.

Condensed Facts: Although used in the past for everything from cancer to respiratory problems, Promensil, which was developed in Australia, was made available in the United States in April 1998. It contains high concentrations of "estrogen-like" (phytoestrogen) compounds called isoflavones.

Conditions: Menopausal symptoms.

Plants/Standard: Usual dosage is 2 to 4 grams of dried flowers up to three times/day.

What to Look For: The preferred product is probably Promensil.

Traditional Dosing/ Dosage Forms: Follow label directions.

Actions/Uses: The active components have estrogen-like actions but are much less potent than estrogen. Therefore, several weeks of therapy may be required prior to experiencing any effects.

Precautions: Not to be used by pregnant or nurs-
                                    ing women, or by those who have a
                                    family history of breast or uterine
                                    cancer.

Typical Price: Tea, 1 oz = $3.50
                                    Tincture, 1 oz = $8.00
                                    Capsules, 90 = $19.00

Soy
Glycine max

Condensed Facts: Soy protein has been shown to be effective in the reduction of blood lipids (high cholesterol). Isoflavone-type chemicals in soy have demonstrated "estrogen-like" (phytoestrogen) activity.

Conditions: Menopausal symptoms.

Plants/Standard: No standards have been established.

What to Look For: Soy can be obtained at grocery stores in the form of fresh or dried beans, tofu, soy milk, etc. These food products are not standardized with respect to their content of phytoestrogens.

Traditional Dosing/ Dosage Forms: See above.

Actions/Uses: Treatment of menopausal symptoms.

Precautions: None known, but there is the potential that these phytoestrogens in very high doses could stimulate estrogen-dependent cancers.

Typical Price: Varies according to the type of product used. Some companies are now selling purified soy protein extracts as well as purified isoflavone mixtures. The prices of these products are significantly higher than the unstandardized soy foods.

Other Herbals for Potential Use to Alleviate Menopause and Menstrual Problems

BUGLE WEED (*Lycopus* spp.)

The aboveground parts of the plant were used as an official drug in the United States from 1830 to 1880. It was used for the treatment of a variety of conditions including hemorrhage, dysentery, and as a sedative. Studies in Europe have confirmed activities that it decreases pituitary sex hormones, thyroid, and prolactin levels. No therapeutic trials have been conducted.

SILVERWEED (*Potentilla anserina* L.)

The dried aboveground parts have a very high tannin content (6 to 10 percent) and thus have been used as an astringent, both internally and externally. Two to 4 grams of plant is used for a tea to treat painful menstruation, diarrhea, or mild inflammation of mouth or throat. May cause irritation of the stomach.

SHEPHERD'S PURSE (*Capsella bursa-pastoris*)

It was used in folk medicine to stop nosebleeds and excessive menstruation. For the latter, a tea of 10 to 15 grams is advised, up to 10 teaspoonfuls!

YARROW (*Achillea millefolium* **L.**)

Milfoil (yarrow) leaves and flowering tops were official drugs in the United States from 1860 to 1880. They were used for menstrual disorders as well as a stimulant and tonic. Europeans now use yarrow primarily for digestive disorders.

Herbal Benefits of Remedies
to Alleviate Menopause
and Menstrual Problems

The use of synthetic or semisynthetic estrogen products is well documented in medical literature to treat various conditions. Some herbals have a long history of use, e.g., black cohosh, chasteberry, and dong quai, whereas recent introductions of natural sources of estrogen-like herbs, such as red clover and soy, have stimulated a resurgence of interest in medicinal plants. Although beneficial effects of soy isoflavones in combination with soy protein on blood cholesterol levels are well documented, the activity of these phytoestrogens with respect to breast or prostate cancer, osteoporosis, or hot flashes requires additional study.

SECTION V:
HERBAL REMEDIES
TO AID PROSTATE HEALTH

Saw Palmetto
Serenoa repens (Barb.) Small

Condensed Facts:

In the older literature, saw palmetto is referred to as sabal. The dried, ripe fruit preparations were used in the past for chest, nose and throat conditions, and "diseases of the glands of reproductive organs."

Conditions:

Benign prostatic hyperplasia (BPH) (non-malignant enlargement of the prostate).

Plants/Standard:

The concentrated extracts of the fruits (berries) yield a mixture of fatty oils, which are assumed to be the active components. Most products contain 85 to 95 percent fatty acids and sterols.

What to Look For:

Products used in clinical trials of over 1,500 male patients used 320 mg/day of the extract. Most products contain this quantity.

Traditional Dosing/ Dosage Forms:

Capsules and/or tablets, alone or in combination with other herbs, although none of the combination products have been shown to be any more effective.

Actions/Uses: An effective agent to be used for the signs and symptoms of BPH. These include difficulty starting urination, weak stream, frequent urination, dribbling, and waking up frequently at night to urinate. Up to four to six weeks of therapy may be required to experience the effects.

Precautions: No significant side effects; a few reports of stomach complaints. No drug interactions. Before beginning self-medication, all people should obtain a professional diagnosis to rule out prostate cancer.

Typical Price: Tincture, 1 oz = $9.00
Capsules and/or tablets,
60 = $19.50

Nettle

Urtica dioica L.

Condensed Facts: The fruit (seeds), leaves, and roots have been used since ancient times for a wide variety of ailments.

Conditions: Limited studies indicate the root may help enlarged prostate problems.

Plants/Standard: Nettle root has not been thoroughly studied to determine which are the active compounds, but sterols and terpenes are probably involved.

What to Look For: Nettle root has not been as extensively studied as saw palmetto; however, twelve clinical trials have yielded positive results for BPH (benign prostatic hyperplasia).

Traditional Dosing/ Dosage Forms: A daily dose of 4 to 6 grams (3 to 5 teaspoonfuls) is usually recommended.

Actions/Uses: Used to increase the volume and flow of urine, and to reduce the amount of residual urine in the bladder.

Precautions:

A study of the safety of nettle root in some 4,000 patients revealed minimal side effects. Less than 1 percent cited stomach problems. However, the dosage (1,200 mg) was below the recommended dose.

Typical Price:

Tincture, 1 oz = $9.00
Capsules, 45 = $9.50 - $11.00
Root powder, 1 oz = $1.50

Pygeum
Prunus africana (Hook. f) Kalkman

Condensed Facts:
The powdered bark of this evergreen tree has many ecologically sensitive people concerned since it is being harvested excessively, and the species may become endangered. Cultivation efforts have begun.

Conditions:
Used for nonmalignant prostate problems.

Plants/Standard:
The bark is made into extracts of varying concentrations.

What to Look For:
One source states that 50 to 100 mg twice a day of an extract that contains 14 percent triterpenes and 0.5 percent *n*-docosanol is effective.

**Traditional Dosing/
Dosage Forms:**
Up to 200 mg/day of an extract has been used in clinical trials.

Actions/Uses:
Used for the treatment of symptoms of BPH including painful urination, frequent night urination, and residual urine in the bladder.

Precautions:
No toxicity has been reported. Once again, as with saw palmetto and

51

others, a thorough diagnosis to exclude prostate cancer should be obtained before self-therapy is begun.

Typical Price: Tincture, 1 oz = $9.00

Other Herbals for Potential Use to Aid Prostate Health

PUMPKIN SEEDS (*Cucurbita pepo* L.)

These have been used as a food source for many years. At least one variety is now known to contain compounds that can alleviate the symptoms of BPH. Usual dose is 1 to 2 tablespoonfuls, well chewed.

RYE (*Secale cereale* L.), TIMOTHY (*Phleum pratense* L.), *AND* CORN (*Zea mays*) POLLEN EXTRACTS

A combination extract studied in two clinical trials of 160 patients showed significant benefits. Doses range from 80 to 120 mg in two to three divided doses for at least three months.

SITOSTEROL-RICH PLANTS (*Hypoxis rooperi*) *AND OTHERS*

Many plants are rich in this compound. It is not a true sterol as found in animals but a sterol very common in plants. *Hypoxis rooperi* has been studied in two clinical trials with positive results. Sitosterol-rich, margarine-like compounds have been recently introduced to reduce cholesterol, similar to a liquid preparation sold over thirty years ago by Eli Lilly and Company (Cytellin).

Herbal Benefits of Remedies to Aid Prostate Health

As with all remedies in this category, one must exclude the possibility that no prostate cancer exists before beginning therapy.

Some drugs that are used to treat prostate problems may lead to the following:

- Cardura—headaches (10 - 14 percent of patients); dizziness (15 - 19 percent)
- Flomax—headaches (19 percent); dizziness (15 percent); runny nose (13 percent)
- Hytrin—headaches (5 percent); dizziness (9 percent)
- Proscar—impotence (8 percent); decreased sexual desire (6 percent); has a failure rate of 26 percent.

To date, no similar adverse reactions have been shown to occur with any of the herbals, especially saw palmetto. Nineteen properly designed clinical studies in nearly 3,000 subjects have documented the effectiveness and essential lack of adverse effects of that herb.

SECTION VI:
HERBAL REMEDIES
TO AID WEIGHT LOSS

Ephedra (Ma Huang)
Ephedra sinica Stapf

Condensed Facts:

The Chinese remedy, ephedra (ma huang), was originally used primarily for its effects on the respiratory system, e.g., congestion, asthma, and coughing.

Conditions:

It is now used in many weight loss products but not without significant adverse effects. Ma huang increases blood pressure and heart rate, and is a central nervous system stimulant. As such, it can cause loss of appetite, but concomitantly causes irritability, insomnia, nausea, flushing, tingling, heart palpitations, and more.

Plants/Standard:

The principal active component, ephedrine, has been used in the United States since the 1930s. Many over-the-counter products contain it or its chemical cousin, pseudoephedrine. Several dietary supplements containing ephedra or ephedrine, often with caffeine-containing herbs, are being marketed as "natural" weight loss aids.

What to Look For:

Ephedra (ma huang) and pseudo-ephedrine products are widely available in nearly all dosage forms. Never take any of these for more than one week.

Traditional Dosing/ Dosage Forms:

Ephedrine dosage is usually 12.5 to 25 mg 3 times/day; pseudoephedrine dosage is 30 to 60 mg 3 times/day. Ma huang tea can be prepared using 1 teaspoonful of dried herb.

Actions/Uses:

Ephedrine is a chemical cousin to adrenaline (epinephrine) and consequently can cause rapid heartbeat, high blood pressure, agitation, insomnia, nausea, and loss of appetite. All of these effects are increased if it is taken together with caffeine. Many states have instituted rules and regulations regarding quantities and strengths that may be legally sold. Excessively high doses have been promoted for use as an "herbal high." To date, thirty-eight deaths due to heart failure from such use have been documented by the FDA.

Precautions:

Individuals with high blood pressure, heart disease, diabetes, glaucoma, hardening of the arteries, thyroid disease, or an enlarged prostate should not take ephedra or anything related to it. Consumption should be limited to adults for a maximum of seven days.

Typical Price: Tincture, 1 oz = $9.00
Powdered herb, 1 oz = $1.00

Other Herbals for Potential Use in the Aid of Weight Loss

FIBER (*Plantago* spp.)
AND OTHER SOURCES

Mentioned in the constipation section, plantago (psyllium) can be used as a bulking agent to decrease appetite. Similar bulking products are now heavily marketed by food and nutritional companies as a means to reduce excessive food consumption, and to lower cholesterol.

OAT BRAN (*Avena sativa*)

Also has been promoted for use to aid in weight loss and to lower cholesterol.

GUAR GUM
[*Cyamopsis tetragonolobus* (L.) Taubert]

Can also be used to aid in weight loss and lowering cholesterol.

Care must be taken to consume large quantities of water with any of these fiber-like products. If these products do not reach the stomach, they can swell higher up in the esophagus with dangerous consequences.

Herbal Benefits of Remedies
to Aid Weight Loss

Nothing can prevent weight gain better than decreasing food consumption and increasing exercise. In the entire range of products from natural ephedrine to synthetic amphetamine-like derivatives (Desoxyn, Meridia), none is without significant adverse effects, especially in higher doses.

SECTION VII:
HERBAL REMEDIES
TO ALLEVIATE HEADACHE/PAIN

Feverfew
Tanacetum parthenium (L.) Schultz Bip.

Condensed Facts:

Feverfew leaves have a long history of multiple uses to treat fever, headache, arthritis, asthma, and digestive disorders. Feverfew is primarily used to treat migraine headaches.

Conditions:

Used primarily for the prevention of chronic, recurrent migraine headaches.

Plants/Standard:

Over fifty-one compounds have been identified. Parthenolide was assumed to be the active chemical and many products were standardized to contain at least 0.2 percent. A recent study has shown that parthenolide may not be the active principle, and most authorities prefer the use of fresh or dried whole leaf preparations.

What to Look For:

Products should contain fresh or dried whole leaf. Stems and root products have not been studied.

Traditional Dosing/ Dosage Forms:

Use 50 to 250 mg of dried feverfew leaves a day; 2½ leaves are approximately equal to 60 mg of dried leaves, therefore, 2 to 10 leaves.

Actions/Uses: Prevention of migraine headache.

Precautions: People allergic to chamomile, rag-
                           weed, or yarrow may be sensitive to
                           feverfew. Not to be used during
                           pregnancy or while breast-feeding.
                           Use with caution if taking with
                           blood-thinning drugs. Otherwise, no
                           reports of toxicity.

Typical Price: Tincture, 1 oz = $9.50
                           Capsules, 60 (100 mg each) = $7.95

Willow Bark
Salix spp.

Condensed Facts:

Salicin-rich species are *S. purpurea* L. (purple osier), *S. daphnoides* (common osier) and *S. fragilis* L. (crack willow).

Conditions:

Used for headaches, rheumatic disorders, or fever.

Plants/Standard:

The barks of different species contain 1.5 to 11 percent of salicin as well as many other compounds.

What to Look For:

Chopped or ground bark used as a tea, tincture, or tablets/capsules.

Traditional Dosing/ Dosage Forms:

Two to 3 grams of bark for a tea (1 teaspoon = 1.5 grams). Capsules are available, but several capsules per day are required to achieve same effect as 500 mg aspirin (acetylsalicylic acid). High concentration of tannins in the bark produce a bitter taste and may cause irritant effects on stomach.

Actions/Uses:

Headache, rheumatic disorders, fever, and anti-inflammatory conditions.

Precautions: None known, but persons with sali-
                          cylate sensitivity should not con-
                          sume.

Typical Price: Tincture, 1 oz = $8.00
                          Capsules, 100 = $10.00

Red Pepper
Capsicum spp.

Condensed Facts: Aside from its use as a spice, the cayenne, paprika, or tobasco pepper can be used for indigestion and stimulating the appetite. However, the topical use is well documented to be effective.

Conditions: Used in creams and ointments for pain relief.

Plants/Standard: Capsaicin is the compound responsible for the "hot" taste in all peppers.

What to Look For: Any approved over-the-counter cream or ointment that contains 0.025 to 0.075 percent capsaicin.

Traditional Dosing/ Dosage Forms: Use as directed.

Actions/Uses: Posthepatic neuralgia, arthritis, and other painful irritations.

Precautions: Do not apply to damaged skin, eyes, or other mucosal tissue.

Typical Price: Cream or ointment, 2 oz = $5.00 depending on strength and manufacturer.

Herbal Benefits of Remedies
to Alleviate Headache/Pain

First came willow bark (*Salix* spp.), then morphine from the opium poppy, then aspirin, then acetaminophen (Tylenol), then ibuprofen (Motrin), and many others.

Aspirin is widely used, but everyone knows its effects, particularly on the stomach. Acetaminophen in overdosage, or in alcohol abusers, can cause liver damage. Ibuprofen can contribute to ulcers and should not be taken for more than seven days. All of these also interact with many other medicines.

In contrast, oral use of feverfew and willow bark have exceedingly low toxicity reports and no known drug-drug interactions. Feverfew is the only known herbal to date with documented evidence that it can prevent or reduce the severity of migraines.

SECTION VIII:
HERBAL REMEDIES
TO ALLEVIATE CONSTIPATION

Aloe

Aloe barbadensis Mill.

Condensed Facts:

The plant is native to Africa but is now widely cultivated in the United States (Florida, Texas, and Arizona). Other species are also used, but current production is mostly of the leaf gel for the cosmetics or beverage industry.

Conditions:

Of all the anthraquinone glycosides, those in aloe are the most potent laxatives. The herb is ten times stronger than rhubarb or senna, and five times stronger than cascara.

Plants/Standard:

Aloe, the laxative, is obtained from cells of the plant near the surface, whereas the gel is obtained from cells found in the central portion of the leaf. Manufacturers that crush the whole leaf for the gel may be processing and selling products with potential laxative effects.

What to Look For:

Aloe products should contain 0.1 to 0.2 grams of aloe, or 0.05 to 0.1 grams of aloe extract. These contain 25 to 40 percent aloins.

Traditional Dosing/ Dosage Forms:	Aloe and the more purified aloins have been used as laxative preparations for years, but due to their excessive stimulation they were replaced by milder laxatives such as rhubarb, senna, and caseara.
Actions/Uses:	Laxative.
Precautions:	Not for use during pregnancy or lactation. Chronic or excessive use may cause potassium loss. Some people may experience a harmless discoloration of the urine.
Typical Price:	Tincture, 1 oz = $5.00 Capsules, 100 = $36.00

Cascara
Rhamnus purshianus

Condensed Facts:

Bark of the tree from the north Pacific Coast states of Washington and Oregon. Bark is stripped from the tree and dried for one year before use.

Conditions:

Cascara is a stimulant laxative due to anthraquinone compounds, which are also found in rhubarb, buckthorn, senna, and aloe. At one time, cascara was one of the most widely used laxatives but was replaced by others. Newer agents such as phenolphthalein and danthron are now in disfavor, and these plant-derived laxatives are again becoming popular, especially senna. According to the FDA, these anthraquinones are no longer approved as drugs because of their mutagenic potential, which is questionable.

Plants/Standard:

Most products contain 20-160 mg of cascarosides.

What to Look For:

Aromatic fluidextract is the best product, usually ½ to 1 teaspoonful

Note: *Rhamnus frangula* L. (buckthorn bark or berries) is a related tree found in Europe, North Africa, and Asia where it is more popular than cascara.

once daily. Tablets (325 mg each) are taken once at bedtime.

Traditional Dosing/ Dosage Forms: Cascara can be used as a tea (½ teaspoonful of powdered herb per cup) taken at bedtime. It is very bitter. It is most often found in a mixture with other agents as a powdered herb, as a fluidextract, or an elixir.

Actions/Uses: It is a highly effective evacuant without excess cramping. It produces a soft stool, which is desirable for persons with anal fissures, hemorrhoids, etc.

Precautions: Not to be used in pregnancy or during lactation. Excess use could result in potassium depletion, causing muscle weakness and heart irregularities. The use of laxatives more than four times per month may be called laxative dependence. This practice should be avoided unless advised by a qualified physician when large doses of constipation medicines are prescribed; for example, in patients taking morphine for cancer pain. A high roughage diet, exercise, and adequate fluid intake should be used instead.

Typical Price: Tea, 1 oz = $0.75
Tincture, 1 oz = $8.00
Capsules, 90 = $8.49

Rhubarb
Rheum spp.

Condensed Facts:
The rhubarb used for a laxative action is not the common garden rhubarb, which is relatively inactive. The plant is a native of western China but may also be imported from Nepal, India, or Pakistan.

Conditions:
Used for treating constipation.

Plants/Standard:
The powdered root is used. The active compounds found in the peeled underground parts range in concentrations from 3 to 12 percent. These also contain 5 to 10 percent tannins, which have the opposite effect, explaining why it is used both as an appetite stimulant and an astringent.

What to Look For:
Rhubarb can be found in bulk at some health stores. It is not currently found in commercially prepared products.

Traditional Dosing/ Dosage Forms:
Can be consumed as a tea (1 to 2 grams dose; 1 teaspoonful = 2 grams). Found in many commercial products, often in combinations, and

has been seen in "diet" remedies, "blood-cleaning cures," and is a component of Swedish bitters.

Actions/Uses:

Because of the varying concentrations of the active components, laxative effects may not be the same. In normal doses and at lower concentrations, a mild laxative effect is produced. However, if the rhubarb product contains more than 12 percent anthracene derivatives, it may cause cramping, colic, and other unwanted actions.

Precautions:

Not to be used during pregnancy or lactation, or if gall bladder problems are present. Chronic use, or overdosage, may deplete potassium in the blood affecting the muscles and the heart.

Typical Price:

Tea, 1 oz = $1.00
Tincture, 1 oz = $8.00

Senna
Cassia spp.

Condensed Facts:

C. angustifolia Vahl is known in commerce as Tinnevelly senna, and *C. senna* L. is known as Alexandria senna. The leaflets are harvested in southern India or the Nile valley, respectively. Both species are now often grouped together as *Senna alexandria* Mill. The leathery seed pods (senna fruit) are also used.

Conditions:

Senna is an effective laxative yielding soft stools, making it beneficial for persons with anal fissures or hemorrhoids, after anal-rectal surgery, or before X-ray examinations.

Plants/Standard:

The leaf contains 2 to 3 percent active ingredients (sennosides), and the pods (fruit) contain 3 to 6 percent. The plant is much less expensive than some others, and therefore is found in many products.

What to Look For:

As with aloe and cascara, senna is still permitted to be sold but is no longer approved by the FDA as a drug because of its mutagenic potential, which is questionable. Found in products such as Senokot, Swiss Kriss, Regular Strength Ex-Lax, and others.

Traditional Dosing/ Dosage Forms:

As a tea, the leaflet is effective in a 1 gram dose (½ teaspoonful) whereas the pods are effective at half that dose (0.5 grams).

Actions/Uses:

Senna is a potent laxative and is very widely used.

Precautions:

Not to be used during pregnancy or lactation. May cause a harmless coloration of the urine. Not to be used chronically or at high doses since potassium depletion may occur, causing muscle weakness and heart irregularities.

Typical Price:

Tea, 1 oz = $0.50
Tincture, 1 oz = $6.00
Capsules, 90 = $12.00

Psyllium

Plantago ovata Forskal, *P. ispagula*

Condensed Facts:

Plantago seeds produce 10 to 12 percent mucilage which, when taken with large volumes of water, causes a laxative effect (bulk laxative). It is a good source of dietary fiber and has been found to reduce cholesterol and low-density lipoprotein (LDL).

Conditions:

Used as a laxative.

Plants/Standard:

The ground, oval, boat-shaped seeds are usually found in prepared products. They contain mucilage.

What to Look For:

Products containing psyllium seed, sometimes called plantaginis. Not to be confused with Plantaginisi herb, which is plantain. Some psyllium products are Konsyl, Metamucil, Perdiem, Reguloid Natural, Serutan, and others.

**Traditional Dosing/
Dosage Forms:**

Not applicable.

Actions/Uses:

The direct stimulation of the bulk formed in the intestine will cause evacuation, usually smoothly because of the mucilage.

Precautions: Not to be used if intestinal obstruction is present.

Typical Price: Capsules, 18 = $12.00
Prepared Products:
     Konsyl
     Metamucil
     Perdiem
     Reguloid Natural
     Serutan

Other Herbals for Potential Use to Alleviate Constipation

COLOCYNTH, JALAP, AND PODOPHYLLUM

All of these plants contain compounds that are extremely potent and are referred to in the medical/pharmacy literature as drastic cathartics. They are used infrequently today, but there is an interesting history of use. In the early 1800s, the Lewis and Clark expedition carried large quantities of podophyllum for laxative purposes. The same plant has yielded chemicals that have been found effective in treating warts, and now has two derivatives that are approved for use in treating breast and cervical cancer. Only podophyllum is found in one commercial laxative preparation. It is available as a resin for removing skin warts (very toxic).

Herbal Benefits of Remedies to Alleviate Constipation

The herbal laxatives, especially psyllium, are the most widely used of all laxative preparations, particularly since the removal of phenolphthalein (the old Ex-Lax active chemical) and danthron from store shelves. The only other stimulant laxative, which is not an herbal, is Dulcolax (bisacodyl), used primarily for bowel cleaning prior to surgery or X-ray examinations.

SECTION IX:
HERBAL REMEDIES
TO ALLEVIATE LIVER DYSFUNCTION

Milk Thistle
Silybum marianum (L.) Gaertn.

Condensed Facts:

The Marian thistle fruit (seed) is now being cultivated due to high demand.

Conditions:

Liver dysfunction ranging from alcoholic cirrhosis to poisonings.

Plants/Standard:

The fruits contain 1.5 to 3.0 percent of a mixture of four compounds called silymarin. Most products contain the equivalent of 200 to 400 mg of silymarin.

What to Look For:

Ground fruits can be found but require doses of 12 to 15 grams/day. It is much more convenient to buy capsules or tincture containing the more purified active compounds.

Traditional Dosing/ Dosage Forms:

It is available as either dried ground fruits, tinctures, or capsules. In Europe, an injectable form is available for medical emergencies (*Amanita* mushroom poisoning). If necessary, the injection can be obtained from the Centers for Disease Control and Prevention in Atlanta, Georgia.

Actions/Uses: For use in toxic liver damage due to poisonings, to treat inflammation, liver conditions, and liver cirrhosis. It does this by two mechanisms:
1. preventing penetration of the poison into the liver cells, and
2. stimulating the formation (regeneration) of new liver cells.

Precautions: None known.

Typical Price: Tincture, 1 oz = $9.00
Capsules, 90 = $15.50
Seeds, 1 oz = $1.75

Schisandra
Schisandra chinensis (Turcz.) Baill.

Condensed Facts: The seeds of schisandra have long been used in China to increase stamina and fight fatigue, and is nowadays used to treat liver ailments.

Conditions: Liver dysfunction.

Plants/Standard: The berries are used, and can be found in Chinese herbal stores or in many Chinese products, usually combined with other herbs. No standards have been established for the yet unknown active compounds. A compound called gomisine may be involved.

What to Look For: Products that are labeled *S. chinensis*.

Traditional Dosing/ Dosage Forms: Follow label directions or the advice of a physician trained in TCM (traditional Chinese medicine).

Actions/Uses: Liver inflammation due to a variety of conditions, e.g., poisoning, hepatitis, jaundice, etc.

Precautions: None known.

Typical Price: Not usually available as a single
                                        ingredient product in the United
                                        States.

Dandelion Root

Taraxacum officinale Weber

Condensed Facts:
Mentioned elsewhere for bladder problems, the root is mentioned frequently by herbalists for liver problems (increases bile flow).

Conditions:
Included in many products to treat bile secretion disorders.

Plants/Standard:
No standards have been established. Unknown active compounds.

What to Look For:
Many phytomedicines are produced in Europe and are now found in the United States which contain dandelion root.

Traditional Dosing/ Dosage Forms:
One to 3 grams of finely chopped root material for a tea. Proprietary products should be taken according to label directions.

Actions/Uses:
Used for bile disorders and digestive complaints. (Some sellers exploit this latter use by putting large quantities of dandelion root in weight loss products.)

Precautions:
Should not be used by those who have a bile duct obstruction (gallstones) or intestinal blockage.

Typical Price: Tincture, 1 oz = $9.00
                                      Capsules, 45 = $9.50
                                      Powder, 1 oz = $1.75

Herbal Benefits of Remedies
to Alleviate Liver Dysfunction

No other medicines, prescription or over-the-counter, exist that have the biological properties of silymarin or schisandra. The potent and proven response of silymarin for use in a variety of liver ailments makes it a remedy without equal.

SECTION X:
HERBAL REMEDIES
TO ALLEVIATE BLADDER PROBLEMS

Goldenrod
Solidago spp.

Condensed Facts: The plant is considered to be an anti-inflammatory diuretic. In folk medicine, it is used as a so-called "blood-purifying" agent for gout, rheumatism, arthritis, as well as eczema and other skin disorders.

Conditions: Used for urinary tract inflammation and to prevent the formation of and to help eliminate kidney stones.

Plants/Standard: Over 130 species are known. Most probably have similar effects. Activity may be due to leiocarposide, a phenolic glycoside, or a saponin, polygalic acid, or various flavonoids. Standardized products are generally not available in the United States.

What to Look For: Goldenrod herb consists of the aboveground parts of the plant, carefully dried.

Traditional Dosing/ Dosage Forms: Use 1 to 1½ teaspoonfuls per cup of water as a tea taken three to five times/day.

Action/Uses: The German Commission E advises that this can be used for prevention and treatment in cases of urinary stones, kidney gravel, and irrigation in cases of inflammation.

Precautions: None known. Should be used with generous amounts of water (six to eight glasses/day). Goldenrod has the undeserved reputation as an allergen because it flowers at the height of the hay fever season. However, most of the hay fever at that time of year is caused by the pollen from the giant ragweed (*Ambrosia* spp.).

Typical Price: Tea, 1 oz = $1.25
                          Tincture, 1 oz = $8.00
                          Capsules, 90 = $19.00

Parsley

Petroselinum crispum (Mill.) A.W. Hill

Condensed Facts:

Parsley root is a milder diuretic than the seeds, although both in higher doses can have negative effects on the intestines, uterus, and liver.

Conditions:

Diuretic (aquaretic), which increases the flow of urine.

Plants/Standard:

The major component is the volatile oil containing apiol and myristicin; oil concentrations vary from 0.1 percent in the roots, 0.3 percent in the leaves, and 2 to 7 percent in the fruits. Standardized preparations are not available in the United States.

What to Look For:

Dried parsley root. Fresh leaves can be dried for tea preparation.

Traditional Dosing/ Dosage Forms:

As a tea, 1 teaspoonful (2 grams) two to three times/day from root material. Not usually found in any products to date since it is available in markets (leaf).

Actions/Uses:

Used for disorders of the urinary tract for prevention and treatment of kidney stones.

Precautions: Not to be used by pregnant women
                                   or persons with a history of easily
                                   sunburned or light skin. Parsley fruit
                                   preparations should not be used dur-
                                   ing pregnancy.

Typical Price: Tea, 1 oz = $1.25
                                   Tincture, 1 oz = $8.00
                                   Capsules, 100 = $10.00

Birch
Betula spp.

Condensed Facts:	*B. pendula* (white or silver birch) or *B. pubescens* (downy birch).
Conditions:	Leaves are used as a diuretic (aquaretic), increasing urine flow.
Plants/Standard:	The plants contain up to 3 percent flavonoids (hyperoside and quercitrin), up to 0.5 percent ascorbic acid (Vitamin C), and various procyanidins. No single component is identified as the active ingredient. Standardized preparations are not generally available.
What to Look For:	Currently there are no standardized products available. One should use the leaves that are collected in spring and dried at room temperature in the shade. They should contain not less than 1.5 percent flavonoids.
Traditional Dosing/ Dosage Forms:	Use as a tea, taking 1 to 1½ grams (1 teaspoonful = 1 gram) two to three times/day. This herb is often found in a mixture in many herbal products, usually as aqueous extracts or in capsules.

Actions/Uses: Used for bacterial and inflammatory conditions of the urinary tract and kidney gravel.

Precautions: None known. Should be taken with generous amounts of water.

Typical Price: Tea, 1 oz = $1.00
                               Tincture, 1 oz = $6.00

Bearberry
Arctostaphylos uva-ursi (L.) Spreng.

Condensed Facts:

Uva-ursi leaf can have urinary anti-septic and astringent effects.

Conditions:

Used as a urinary antiseptic in mild conditions, not a diuretic. It requires an alkaline urine for best effect. One way to do so is to take sodium bicarbonate (baking soda), ½ teaspoonful in 4 fl oz of water every two hours. Caution should be exercised in persons who cannot consume large sodium doses, for example persons with high blood pressure, diabetes, etc.

Plants/Standard:

The principal active compound is arbutin, which is absorbed and then converted in the body to hydroquinone, a compound known for its antiseptic properties. It was widely used from 1820 until 1950 when other products became available, such as the oral sulfanilamides.

What to Look For:

Products should contain not less than 5 percent arbutin, a hydroquinone glycoside derivative.

Traditional Dosing/ Dosage Forms:

When used as a tea, 2 to 10 grams (1 to 5 teaspoonfuls), preferably made by steeping in cold water to avoid removing excess bitter substances (tannins). Found in tea bags in Europe and diet supplements in the United States, usually as a mixture with other herbal diuretics such as buchu, birch, etc.

Actions/Uses:

Inflammatory conditions of the urinary tract.

Precautions:

Not to be used during pregnancy, lactation, or in children under twelve years old. Do not take for extended periods of time. Do not take at the same time as Vitamin C or cranberry products. These products can produce acidic urine and decrease the effectiveness of uva ursi.

Typical Price:

Tea, 1 oz = $1.50
Tincture, 1 oz = $8.00
Capsules, 90 = $19.00

Cranberry
Vaccinium macrocarpon Ait.

Condensed Facts:

Primarily considered a food source, cranberry juice has been used in traditional medicine as a diuretic, antiseptic, and antipyretic.

Conditions:

Uncomplicated urinary tract infections (UTI). It works by preventing harmful bacteria from "sticking" to the surface of the cells in the urinary tract so they can than be removed by the urine.

Plants/Standard:

The ripe berries contain condensed tannins (oligomeric proanthocyanidins) that are believed to be the principal active ingredients. Standardized products are not available.

What to Look For:

Concentrated cranberry extract tablets or capsules are available (usually 400 mg).

Traditional Dosing/ Dosage Forms:

Cranberry juice cocktail is usually consumed at 3 to 16 or more oz/day. It consists of about one-third pure juice. Capsules are also available containing the powdered (non-extracted) berries.

Actions/Uses:	Prevention of urinary tract infections.
Precautions:	None known.
Typical Price:	Capsules, 90 = $11.99

Other Herbals for Potential
Use to Alleviate Bladder Problems

LOVAGE (*Levisticum officinale* W.D. J. Koch)

Roots are used, 1 to 3 teaspoonfuls as a tea. May increase sensitivity to sunburn.

JUNIPER (*Juniperus communis* L.)

Berries are used, ¾ teaspoonful. Not to be used during pregnancy or by persons with kidney problems.

DANDELION (*Taraxacum officinale* Weber)

Leaves are used (1 to 2½ teaspoonfuls daily) for bladder problems. The root is used to stimulate liver function and as an appetite stimulant.

COUCH-GRASS (*Triticum repens*)

Roots, rhizomes, and stems are used. Also used as a cough remedy. As a tea, 5 to 10 grams/day (1 teaspoonful = 1.5 grams, therefore, 3 to 7 teaspoonfuls).

Note: Most of these herbs are listed in books on folklore use and based on traditional uses. To date, there has been very little scientific research to document their effectiveness.

Herbal Benefits of Remedies
to Alleviate Bladder Problems

Most of the herbal remedies, with one exception, i.e., cranberry, are used either to stimulate urine flow or fight inflammation of the urinary tract. Cranberry is known to prevent recurrent urinary tract infections. The most widely used anti-infective prescription agents are sulfa-based (Bactrim, Septra) or quinolone derivatives (NegGram), both with very long lists of adverse reactions, contraindications, and precautions.

SECTION XI:
HERBAL REMEDIES
TO ALLEVIATE ULCERS
AND INTESTINAL PROBLEMS

Licorice
Glycyrrhiza glabra L.

Condensed Facts:

Used since ancient times, this shrub is native to the Mediterranean and is now cultivated in Russia, Turkey, and China. The root is used both as a flavor and a medicine.

Conditions:

Used to treat bronchial congestion and stomach and duodenal ulcers. Some herbalists advise use for a wide variety of other conditions, from chronic fatigue syndrome to viral infections. All of these uses are poorly documented.

Plants/Standard:

Licorice contains 2 to 15 percent of glycyrrhizin and related compounds, some of which are 50 to 100 times as sweet as sugar. More than thirty flavonoids have been identified.

What to Look For:

Some products contain deglycyrrhizinated licorice, supposedly to reduce the steroid-like side effects including sodium and water retention, and potassium loss. There are few data to support the contention that these products have the same effects as the whole plant product.

Traditional Dosing/ Dosage Forms: Most licorice-like products (foods, candies, etc.) sold in the United States contain anise, not licorice. Read labels carefully. Licorice tea uses ½ teaspoonful/cup with a four to six week treatment maximum. Extracts with lower concentrations may be consumed for a longer time.

Actions/Uses: Effective for a variety of localized conditions, but use for ulcers has diminished since the discovery that many are bacterial ulcers and can be cured with a short course of antibiotics.

Precautions: Prolonged use or high doses can cause sodium and water retention, and potassium loss with consequent high blood pressure, swelling, or muscle weakness.

Typical Price: Tincture, 1 oz = $9.00
Capsules, 60 = $13.80
Root, 1 oz = $1.75

Ginger
Zingiber officinale Roscoe

Condensed Facts: Many commercial varieties are available from most tropical countries for use in herbals and foods. Now commonly found in garden nurseries because of its vibrant foliage. The active constituents vary widely depending on the source.

Conditions: Used initially as a spice, early Greeks and Romans used it for stomach disorders. Early books found it to be used as a "corrective for nauseous conditions" and hence its current use for dizziness and motion sickness.

Plants/Standard: Use the fresh ground rhizome (underground stem) which has a characteristic aromatic fragrance. Long storage changes the composition of the constituents greatly.

What to Look For: Products such as powdered ginger, ginger tea, and some European extracts in tablets or capsules are available. No standards established.

Traditional Dosing/ Dosage Forms: Average daily dose is approximately 2 grams ($^2/_3$ teaspoonful) up to 4 grams daily, which can be taken in divided doses. Take 1 gram thirty minutes before traveling.

Actions/Uses:

Can be used for stomach complaints but most of the use today is for motion sickness or nausea.

Precautions:

None known. Test tube experiments have shown inhibition by blood coagulation, but three European studies in patients failed to show such an effect.

Typical Price:

Tincture, 1 oz = $9.00
Capsules, 45 = $9.50
Powdered herb, 1 oz = $2.50

Artichoke
Cynara scolymus

Condensed Facts: Europeans have long used artichoke as a food delicacy, but they have also used it for liver disease, indigestion, anemia, and atherosclerosis.

Conditions: Used primarily for its capability to stimulate bile output (choleretic). Thus it can decrease bloating, nausea, and vomiting associated with poor fat absorption. Laboratory animal studies indicate it may have liver protectant properties, similar to silymarin (see Section IX).

Plants/Standard: The leaves contain cynarin and other bitter principles. Most companies standardize to these quinic acid derivatives, usually 15 mg per capsule. The crude leaves can be consumed in doses of 6 grams.

What to Look For: Plant products standardized to contain cynarin.

Traditional Dosing/ Dosage Forms: Capsules, tablets, or tinctures standardized to cynarin content.

Actions/Uses: The most reliable clinical studies to date document the bile-stimulating properties. However, more studies in the future will probably show other uses.

Precautions:　　　　None known to date.

Typical Price:　　　　Tincture, 1 oz = $12.00
Capsules, 60 = $14.95

Other Herbals for Potential Use to Alleviate Ulcers and Intestinal Problems

MARSHMALLOW LEAF OR ROOT
(*Althea officinalis* L.)

Has been used for mild inflammation of the digestive, pulmonary, and mucous membranes due to its mucilage content. Approximately 2 grams of leaf (1 heaping teaspoonful), or 1 to 3 teaspoonfuls of root can be used for a tea.

PEPPERMINT (*Mentha* × *piperita* L.)

Leaf tea and its extracted oils have been used since ancient times for stomach complaints ranging from cramps and spasms to gall bladder problems. One tablespoonful of leaf yields a fragrant tea. An average of 6 to 12 drops of the oil is utilized.

CHAMOMILE (*Matricaria recutita* L.)

Has been mentioned elsewhere (see Section XII), but it is capable of alleviating gastrointestinal spasms and inflammation. One tablespoonful of flowers for a tea, three to four times/day, between meals.

Herbal Benefits of Remedies
to Alleviate Ulcers
and Intestinal Problems

Dyspepsia, a discomfort of the stomach area commonly called indigestion, with localized pain, gasiness, and/or a full, bloated feeling has plagued mankind for years. Antacids, at least 40 brands, have been the mainstay for self-therapy. Many prescription and now nonprescription products (Pepcid, Tagamet, Zantac) were favorites prior to the finding that some true ulcers could be cured with a short course of specific antibiotic therapy. As a result, these products are now used extensively for heartburn and acid indigestion.

Once again, nature provides effective relief for non-ulcer-caused dyspepsia, usually dosed in the form of pleasant-tasting teas, and all without significant side effects when used properly (licorice), and no known interactions with any other medicines.

SECTION XII:
HERBAL REMEDIES
TO ALLEVIATE SKIN PROBLEMS
AND EXTERNAL SORES

Witch Hazel
Hamamelis virginiana L.

Condensed Facts:

The shrub is native to the eastern United States and has been introduced to Europe where it is popular as a winter flowering garden plant. Both the leaves and bark are used.

Conditions:

Used for local skin inflammation and mucous membranes, including hemorrhoids.

Plants/Standard:

The leaf contains 3 to 10 percent tannins; the bark usually contains 10 percent.

What to Look For:

Witch hazel extracts (water) are available but usually contain little or no active compounds. Varies by manufacturer.

Traditional Dosing/ Dosage Forms:

About 2 grams of bark (1 teaspoonful) or 1 to 2 grams of leaf (2 to 4 teaspoonfuls) can make a tea for use as a mouthwash or applied as a poultice (wetted gauze).

Actions/Uses:

Topical anti-inflammatory.

Precautions:

None known.

Typical Price:

Tincture, 1 oz = $9.00
Bark, 1 oz = $1.50

Chamomile
Matricaria recutita L.
or *Chamaemelum nobile* (L.) All.

Condensed Facts:
Matricaria recutita (German chamomile) or *Chamaemelum nobile* (Roman chamomile). Used by ancient Egyptians, Greeks, and Romans for fevers, kidney, liver, and bladder disorders.

Conditions:
Topical use for skin inflammation, but also used as a tea for gastrointestinal problems.

Plants/Standard:
Chamaemelum contain 0.6 to 2.4 percent of the volatile oil, *Matricaria* 0.3 to 1.5 percent.

What to Look For:
Use recently dried flower heads. Proprietary preparations available in Europe, generally not available in the United States to date.

Traditional Dosing/ Dosage Forms:
Use 1 to 2 grams of flowers (1 teaspoonful) for a tea. Some poor quality tea products may contain the whole plant (leaves and stems) and not just the flower.

Actions/Uses: Used as anti-inflammatory, both top-ically and internally.

Precautions: None known.

Typical Price: Tincture, 1 oz = $9.00
Capsules, 45 (1 oz each) = $9.50
Dried flowers, 1 oz = $2.25

Calendula
Calendula officinalis L.

Condensed Facts About: An official drug in the United States from 1880 to 1910 and used since ancient times to heal wounds and treat inflamed skin. Also known as garden marigold.

Conditions: Used for nonhealing skin wounds, inflammation, and hemorrhoids.

Plants/Standard: Contains a wide variety of volatile oils, flavonoids, and triperpene alcohols. Hydroalcoholic extracts (water and alcohol) seem to be the most effective.

What to Look For: Marigold is found in many topical lotions, creams, and ointments, but concentrations vary greatly.

Traditional Dosing/ Dosage Forms: A tea (1 to 2 teaspoonfuls) can be made to use as a poultice and is applied several times per day. Ointments are available in Europe and some now in the United States. Cosmetic manufacturers include *Calendula* frequently.

Actions/Uses: Wound healing.

Precautions: No adverse effects have been re-
                                    ported.

Typical Price: Tea, 1 oz = $2.50
                                    Tincture, 1 oz = $9.00
                                    Capsules, 90 = $19.00

Tea Tree
Melaleuca spp.

Condensed Facts: Captain Cook, following his visit to the South Seas, introduced tea tree leaves to England as a substitute for regular tea. It has since been discovered to have strong antiseptic properties.

Conditions: The oil is used topically for a wide variety of skin conditions, from minor localized irritations to fungal and bacterial infections.

Plants/Standard: The products that are available have a range of oil concentration, from 1 to 100 percent. The lowest concentrations should be employed initially due to the skin irritation that may occur with higher concentrations.

What to Look For: Several manufacturers make a wide variety of soaps, lotions, ointments, mouthwashes, toothpastes, etc.

Traditional Dosing/ Dosage Forms: Topical use only.

Actions/Uses: Used as an antiseptic for many skin conditions.

Precautions: Do not take internally since safety evaluations for such use have not been completed to date.

Typical Price: Varies greatly according to product and concentration of the oil in the product.

Other Herbals for Potential
Use to Alleviate Skin Problems
and External Sores

ARNICA (*Arnica montana* L. and other spp.)

Not for oral use. Used topically for sprains, bruising, rheumatic conditions of joints and muscles, and hematomas. Can be applied as a poultice from tea (2 grams/100 ml of water), a tincture diluted three to ten times with water, or an ointment (maximum 15 percent arnica oil).

COMFREY (*Symphytum officinale* L.)

Not for oral use. Liver-toxic chemicals may also be carcinogenic, with highest concentrations in the roots. Used for sprains, contusions, and bruises in the form of ointments containing 5 to 20 percent of the dried herb.

CONEFLOWER (*Echinacea* spp.)

Aside from other uses, echinacea preparations containing 15 percent or more of the juice from the aboveground parts can be applied topically for treating poorly healing wounds.

Herbal Benefits of Remedies to Alleviate Skin Problems and External Sores

Visit any cosmetic department and notice the large number of choices of products for treating various skin conditions. Labels show that many contain over thirty or more synthetic chemicals.

Nature has provided safe, effective plants that can be prepared easily for conditions ranging from minor skin irritations to documented bacterial and fungal infections. Most herbal products are much less expensive, easy to prepare, safe, and effective.

Index

THE HAWORTH HERBAL PRESS
Varro E. Tyler, PhD
Executive Editor

TYLER'S TIPS: THE SHOPPER'S GUIDE FOR HERBAL REMEDIES by George H. Constantine (2000). "George Constantine has given us a commonsense, easily read, well-organized shopper's guide to the most frequently utilized and best-documented herbal remedies." *Paul L. Schiff Jr., PhD, Professor of Pharmaceutical Sciences, School of Pharmacy, University of Pittsburgh, Pennsylvania*

HANDBOOK OF PSYCHOTROPIC HERBS: A SCIENTIFIC ANALYSIS OF HERBAL REMEDIES FOR PSYCHIATRIC CONDITIONS by Ethan B. Russo (2000). "Sound advice on the rational use of safe and effective herbs to help alleviate a wide range of neurological disorders. An authoritative guide in an area where solid, reliable information is often difficult to obtain." *Mark Blumenthal, Founder and Executive Director, American Botanical Council; Editor,* HerbalGram; *Senior Editor,* The Complete German Commission E Monographs

UNDERSTANDING ALTERNATIVE MEDICINE: NEW HEALTH PATHS IN AMERICA by Lawrence Tyler (2000). "An eye-opening account of the emerging health paths in the United States and other parts of the Western world." *Mark Bender, Assistant Professor of Chinese, Department of East Asian Languages and Literatures, The Ohio State University, Columbus*

SEASONING SAVVY: HOW TO COOK WITH HERBS, SPICES, AND OTHER FLAVORINGS by Alice Arndt (1999). "Well-written and wonderfully comprehensive exploration of the world of herbs, spices and aromatics—at once authorative and easy to use." *Nancy Harmon Jenkins, Author of* The Mediterranean Diet Cookbook

TYLER'S HONEST HERBAL: A SENSIBLE GUIDE TO THE USE OF HERBS AND RELATED REMEDIES, Fourth Edition by Steven Foster and Varro E. Tyler (1999). "An up-to-date revision of the most reliable source for the layperson on herbal medicines. Excellent as a starting point for scientists who desire more information on herbal medicines." *Norman R. Farnsworth, PhD, Research Professor of Pharmacognosy, College of Pharmacy, University of Illinois at Chicago*

TYLER'S HERBS OF CHOICE: THE THERAPEUTIC USE OF PHYTOMEDICINALS, Second Edition by James E. Robbers and Varro E. Tyler (1999). "The first edition of this book was a landmark publication. . . . This new edition will no doubt become one of the most often-used references by health practitioners of all types." *Mark Blumenthal, Founder and Executive Director, American Botanical Council; Editor,* Herbalgram

Order Your Own Copy of
This Important Book for Your Personal Library!

TYLER'S TIPS
The Shopper's Guide for Herbal Remedies

_____ in hardbound at $39.95 (ISBN: 0-7890-0948-X)

_____ in softbound at $14.95 (ISBN: 0-7890-0949-8)

COST OF BOOKS_____

OUTSIDE USA/CANADA/
MEXICO: ADD 20%_____

POSTAGE & HANDLING_____
(US: $4.00 for first book & $1.50
for each additional book
Outside US: $5.00 for first book
& $2.00 for each additional book)

SUBTOTAL_____

IN CANADA: ADD 7% GST_____

STATE TAX_____
(NY, OH & MN residents, please
add appropriate local sales tax)

FINAL TOTAL_____
(If paying in Canadian funds,
convert using the current
exchange rate. UNESCO
coupons welcome.)

☐ **BILL ME LATER:** ($5 service charge will be added)
(Bill-me option is good on US/Canada/Mexico orders only;
not good to jobbers, wholesalers, or subscription agencies.)

☐ Check here if billing address is different from
shipping address and attach purchase order and
billing address information.

Signature_____

☐ **PAYMENT ENCLOSED:** $_____

☐ **PLEASE CHARGE TO MY CREDIT CARD.**

☐ Visa   ☐ MasterCard   ☐ AmEx   ☐ Discover
☐ Diner's Club   ☐ Eurocard   ☐ JCB

Account # _____

Exp. Date _____

Signature _____

Prices in US dollars and subject to change without notice.

NAME _____

INSTITUTION _____

ADDRESS _____

CITY _____

STATE/ZIP _____

COUNTRY _____ COUNTY (NY residents only) _____

TEL _____ FAX _____

E-MAIL_____

May we use your e-mail address for confirmations and other types of information? ☐ Yes   ☐ No
We appreciate receiving your e-mail address and fax number. Haworth would like to e-mail or fax special
discount offers to you, as a preferred customer. **We will never share, rent, or exchange your e-mail
address or fax number.** We regard such actions as an invasion of your privacy.

Order From Your Local Bookstore or Directly From

The Haworth Press, Inc.

10 Alice Street, Binghamton, New York 13904-1580 • USA

TELEPHONE: 1-800-HAWORTH (1-800-429-6784) / Outside US/Canada: (607) 722-5857

FAX: 1-800-895-0582 / Outside US/Canada: (607) 772-6362

E-mail: getinfo@haworthpressinc.com

PLEASE PHOTOCOPY THIS FORM FOR YOUR PERSONAL USE.

www.HaworthPress.com

BOF00